Table of Contents

Introduction

I had been struggling with my health for years, but it wasn't until I was diagnosed with an autoimmune disorder that I finally decided to take control of my life and make a change. After extensive research, I decided to give the autoimmune diet a try.

At first, I was a bit overwhelmed. I had to completely overhaul my diet and eliminate many of the foods I had been accustomed to eating. I had to learn how to read labels, identify inflammatory ingredients, and choose foods that would support my body. It certainly wasn't easy, but I was determined to make the diet work.

The changes I made to my diet were difficult at first, but I soon started to see results. Within a few weeks, I noticed a big improvement in my energy levels and overall well-being. I was also sleeping better, and my digestion and skin health had improved significantly.

As time passed, I continued to make positive changes in my life and my health continued to improve. I was able to reduce the amount of medication I was taking and regained some of the energy I had lost. I was even able to start exercising again and felt stronger than ever.

The autoimmune diet was a huge turning point in my life. I finally felt like I was in control of my health, and I was no longer a slave to my autoimmune disorder. Not only did I feel better than ever, but I also felt empowered and inspired to take on life's challenges.

I'm so thankful for the autoimmune diet and all the positive changes it's helped me make in my life. It's truly changed my life for the better, and

I'm excited to see what else I can accomplish now that I'm living my best life.

Auto immune diet cookbook

LEMON & ASPARAGUS CHICKEN SKILLET

Sometimes you just need an easy one pan meal! I love cooking skillet meals on busy weeknights or for simple meal prep. It helps keep dishes at a minimum and can reduce overall cooking time. I never really took advantage of one pan meals until I started blogging, and now I can't get enough of them. There are so many possibilities for what you can make in one pan, and this lemon & asparagus chicken skillet is a light, fresh and flavorful option.

This one-pan meal comes together in under 45 minutes and uses seasonal ingredients like asparagus, and easy to find protein like chicken breast. It features lemon juice to give it a kick of acid, and just a bit of coconut aminos to give a bit more umami.

Plus, this meal is allergen friendly and is made without any of the common allergens. It's paleo, whole30, and AIP compliant, and great for sharing with family or friends who have gluten, dairy, or soy allergies.

HOW TO MAKE THE LEMON & ASPARAGUS CHICKEN SKILLET RECIPE

Cook the chicken: Add the chicken to the skillet and lightly season with salt and pepper. Cook until the chicken reaches an internal temperature of 165 F.

Cook & prepare the asparagus: Prepare the asparagus by chopping off the thick white base and then slice in half again. Add more oil to the pan if needed and saute the asparagus with more salt and pepper for about 5-7 minutes or until softened and lightly crisp. Set aside.

Combine the chicken & asparagus and make the sauce: Add the broth, lemon juice, coconut aminos, and arrowroot starch to the pan and stir for about 2-3 minutes or until the sauce lightly thickens. Add the chicken and asparagus back to the pan and cook for another 2 minutes to reheat.

THE INGREDIENTS YOU'LL NEED FOR THE LEMON & ASPARAGUS CHICKEN SKILLET

Chicken breast

Either chicken breast or thigh will work for this recipe, but I like using chicken breast! Simply cube it up and you're good to go. This helps it cook a bit faster, and make the meal easier to eat on the go.

Asparagus

Asparagus is really simple to prep and store. What I like to do to store it is to place the bottom of the spears in a mug or glass cup and fill it with about half an inch of water. This helps keep the asparagus fresh and crisp! I've had success with keeping it like this for 3-4 days. From there, you want to cut off about an inch of the thicker base of the spears. With this recipe, you'll cut them in half, but you could easily roast them whole in other recipes like this.

Garlic, green onion, salt, and pepper

You can leave out the pepper if you're AIP, but these flavors help round out the dish.

Lemon juice

The flavor of lemon and asparagus pair really well together, and I love how it tastes in this dish. It's light while still adding a kick with the acid. Fresh lemon juice works best, but refrigerated will work as well.

Chicken broth, coconut aminos, and arrowroot starch

These make a light sauce to add more flavor to the dish and keep it from being dry. The coconut aminos is a soy sauce substitute, and the arrowroot starch works to help thicken the sauce.

INGREDIENTS

2 tbsp avocado oil

1 tsp sea salt, divided

1/2 tsp pepper, divided (omit for AIP)

1 lb chicken breast, cubed

1 bunch asparagus

3 cloves garlic, minced

1/3 cup chicken broth

Juice of one lemon

1 tbsp coconut aminos

1 tsp arrowroot starch

2 tbsp green onion, chopped

INSTRUCTIONS

Using a large skillet, heat the avocado oil on medium heat.

Add the chicken to the skillet and lightly season with salt and pepper. Cook until the chicken reaches an internal temperature of 165 F. Set aside.

Prepare the asparagus by chopping off the thick white base, and then slice in half again.

Add more oil to the pan if needed and saute the asparagus with more salt and pepper for about 5-7 minutes or until softened and lightly crisp. Set aside.

Reduce the heat slightly and add the minced garlic to the pan. Cook until fragrant.

Add the broth, lemon juice, coconut aminos, and arrowroot starch to the pan and stir for about 2-3 minutes or until the sauce lightly thickens.

Add the chicken and asparagus back to the pan and cook for another 2 minutes to reheat.

Serve topped with green onion and season further to taste.

NUTRITION

serving size: 1 SERVINGcalories: 335fat: 15Gcarbohydrates: 14Gfiber: 1.6Gprotein: 36.9G

EASY EGG ROLL IN A BOWL

When it comes to any takeout, I feel like everyone is always down for adding egg rolls to their order. Or at least that's how I got acquainted with a love of egg rolls growing up. My little brother was always asking for them, and who could blame him? Who doesn't love a crispy and flavorful egg roll?

I haven't had an egg roll in years since I've gone grain-free. I completely put them out of my mind... until I became acquainted with the idea of an egg roll in a bowl. All of the flavor of egg rolls but without the fried wrapper! That why I decided to make and AIP, Whole30, keto, and Paleo version of an Egg Roll in a Bowl featuring a ginger cream sauce.

I know what you might be thinking... what's an egg roll without the wrapper? And I hear you! But this dish has so much to offer, if not more, for being made without the wrapper. Really, this meal is all just good quality veggies, protein, healthy fats, and a yummy sauce. It's the perfect dish to cover all of your bases and is a great dinner to batch cook and have for leftovers for lunch!

Egg roll in a bowl with cream sauce

HOW TO MAKE EGG ROLL IN A BOWL

In a large skillet, brown the pork on medium heat and lightly season with salt and pepper. Set aside and discard the fat.

Using the same skillet, heat the oil on medium heat. Saute the onion, garlic, and ginger until fragrant and the onion is translucent.

Pour in the coleslaw mix as well as the apple cider vinegar, coconut aminos. Saute for 4-5 minutes or until the cabbage reduces in size and the carrots soften.

Reincorporate the cooked pork and stir to combine. Saute for another minute to reheat.

Remove from heat and top with green onion and optional garlic cream sauce,

EGG ROLL IN A BOWL TIPS & TRICKS

Make it on the weekend and use it as meal prep for the week!

This egg roll in a bowl is perfect for batch cooking! Make it on Sunday and store it in separate

Tupperware containers to make a quick and easy grab and go lunch. Serve the sauce on the side if you plan to meal prep it.

Mix up the proteins

Don't want to use pork? That's a-okay! This recipe is totally flexible. You can use ground chicken thigh, ground turkey, or even ground beef.

Get creative with the sauces and spices

Like a little more heat? Add some compliant sriracha sauce or some chili flakes. These are not AIP compliant, but they

TO MAKE THIS A KETO EGG ROLL IN A BOWL...

Be careful with the carrots

Make sure you don't use a coleslaw mix that has a ton of carrots as it may be too much sugar.

Double-check your coconut aminos

Some have more sugar than others.

THE INGREDIENTS YOU NEED FOR THE EGG ROLL IN A BOWL

Coleslaw mix

Grab a prepped coleslaw mix at the store that features shredded green cabbage, red cabbage, and shredded carrots for a short cut. If this isn't accessible for you, you can easily buy these ingredients separately.

White and green onion

White onion is in the base, and green onion is used as a garnish.

Ground pork (or other protein)

Pork is what I'm used to in an egg roll, but you can easily swap out something like ground beef, chicken, or even turkey.

Sesame oil (or coconut)

You can easily sub coconut oil if you're AIP!

Ginger, garlic, salt, and pepper

These add the classic flavors that you would find with an egg roll. Omit the pepper for AIP.

Apple cider vinegar and coconut aminos

You can also use rice wine vinegar if you tolerate it. Coconut aminos is the soy sauce substitute.

For the sauce...

For the sauce, you'll need coconut cream, coconut aminos, ginger, salt, and apple cider vinegar.

INGREDIENTS

For The Egg Roll In a Bowl

1 lb ground pork

2 tbsp sesame oil (or coconut oil for AIP)

1 white onion, diced

2 cloves garlic, minced

1 tsp grated ginger

12 oz coleslaw mix

2 tsp apple cider vinegar

3 tbsp coconut aminos

2 tbsp green onion, chopped

For the sauce (optional)

1/4 cup coconut cream

1 tbsp coconut aminos

1 tsp apple cider vinegar

2 tsp fresh ginger, grated

Pinch of sea salt

INSTRUCTIONS

For the egg roll in a bowl

In a large skillet, brown the pork on medium heat and lightly season with salt and pepper. Once cooked, set aside. Discard the fat.

Using the same skillet, heat the oil on medium heat. Saute the onion, garlic and ginger until fragrant and the onion is translucent.

Pour in the coleslaw mix as well as the apple cider vinegar, coconut aminos. Season with the remainder of salt and pepper. Stir well to combine. Saute for 4-5 minutes or until the cabbage reduces in size and the carrots soften.

Reincorporate the cooked pork and stir to combine. Saute for another minute to reheat.

Remove from heat and topped with green onion and optional sauce (see below).

For the optional sauce

Combine all of the ingredients in a bowl and whisk together. Serve over the bowls.

NUTRITION

serving size: 1 SERVINGcalories: 351fat: 15.8Gcarbohydrates: 15.8Gfiber: 2.6Gprotein: 38.2G

Autoimmune diseases are conditions where the body cannot differentiate its own healthy proteins, from the proteins of foreign invaders. The body then attacks its own tissue, causing a hypersensitivity reaction known as an "autoimmune response." This self-tissue attack can go on for months or years before an autoimmune disease fully develops, causing damage to cells, tissues, and/or organs. According to the American Autoimmune Related Diseases Association, autoimmune diseases affect up to 50 million Americans. The type of proteins or cells being attacked is what distinguishes one AI disorder from another

The Autoimmune Protocol (AIP) focuses on reducing inflammation in the gut that causes an autoimmune response. The AIP diet works to calm and decrease inflammation, thereby lessening the disease's symptoms and ideally putting it into remission.

The AIP diet removes: Dairy, Eggs, Legumes, Sugar and high-glycemic foods, Nuts and nut oils, Seeds and seed oils, Spices derived from seeds, Nightshades, Alcohol, Coffee, and Chocolate.

Diet and lifestyle can play a large role in keeping AI diseases under control. By eliminating inflammatory foods, you can create an environment to heal your body from within.

AIP Flatbread

– Healing Autoimmune

AIP Flatbread

Ingredients: coconut flour, cassava flour, baking powder, garlic powder, mixed dried herbs, salt, Nutritional Yeast Flakes, water, gelatin powder, olive oil.

Making bread that fits with your autoimmune diet can be a real problem, but that's where flatbread can be the answer. The one in this recipe has a slightly cheesy flavor because of the nutritional yeast flakes and this would be great to serve with salads or even with soups. You can even change the herbs you use, depending on what you are serving it with.

AIP Waffles

– Healing Autoimmune

Ingredients: gelatin, water, cassava flour, coconut flour, cream of tartar, baking soda, salt, coconut oil, honey, blueberries.

Believe it or not, these waffles are really like regular ones with the same spongy texture, but they are compliant with the autoimmune protocol and can be served for breakfast or a tasty lunch. I like to pair these with some fresh berries for a light but filling breakfast, but you could even dress them up and use them as dessert!

Healing Autoimmune

AIP Coconut Shrimp and Grits

Ingredients: olive oil, button mushrooms, garlic, shrimp, lemon juice, coconut cream, coconut, salt.

Traditional grits are made using corn, but as that is a definite no-no on the AIP this clever recipe uses desiccated coconut to form the grits instead. Although the flavor is different, the texture is the same and this pairs well with the shrimp. You can either use fresh shrimp or thawed frozen ones which are a bit cheaper.

Blueberry Coconut Yogurt Smoothie

– Paleo Flourish

Blueberry Coconut Yogurt Smoothie

Ingredients: coconut yogurt, blueberries, coconut milk.

If you like smoothies but don't fancy the banana-based ones as they can contain extra sugars, then a coconut yogurt-based one can solve the problem! With the natural sweetness from the berries, this drink makes a fresh and fruity start to the day, or a lovely refreshing snack. This recipe could also be used to make an AIP frozen yogurt dessert!

Passion Fruit Coconut Yogurt Parfait

– Paleo Flourish

Passion Fruit Coconut Yogurt Parfait

Ingredients: coconut yogurt, passion fruit, blueberries.

If you are a fan of yogurt but can't have dairy, coconut yogurt could be the answer as it is dairy free. The totally tropical flavor of the passion fruit gives this dish a fantastic summery taste. For strict AIP you'll want to leave off the nuts and seeds. This would be a great dish to make for breakfast because it is so quick to prepare but would also be fine for dessert.

Banana Pancakes

– Paleo Flourish

Banana Pancakes

Ingredients: bananas, coconut flour, baking soda, coconut oil, raw honey or maple syrup, gelatin, water.

As these pancakes are both nut free and grain free, they are ideal for people whose system needs a gentler approach to breakfast. The banana is a great source of magnesium and tastes great. It also releases energy slower than other fruits, so keeps you going till lunch! Compliant with the autoimmune protocol, these pancakes are lovely any time of day.

Sweet Potato Breakfast Hash

– Paleo Flourish

Sweet Potato Breakfast Hash

Ingredients: sweet potato, zucchini, leftover meat, fresh thyme leaves or dried thyme or other herbs of your choosing, coconut oil, salt.

Serving hash for a healthy AIP breakfast can really set you up for the day as it is filling and satisfying and very, very tasty. This hash has a sweet note from the potato, which complements your choice of meat left over from a previous meal. This recipe is gluten free and also suitable for the paleo diet.

Lemon Fried Avocado

– Paleo Flourish

Lemon Fried Avocado

Ingredients: avocado, coconut oil, lemon juice, salt.

Most of us would never have thought of frying avocado slices, but these are amazing with a little lemon juice drizzled over them. They are the perfect AIP-friendly side dish to serve with fish or you could even scatter them over a salad. Try to use avocados that are not too ripe so they will hold their shape while they are cooking.

Garlic & Lemon Wilted Chard

– Autoimmune Wellness

Ingredients: swiss chard, olive oil, garlic, lemon juice, sea salt.

If you are not a confident cook or a total novice in the kitchen, recipes like this one which describes how to cook a vegetable can be very helpful. Chard is a really healthy veg that has quite a strong flavor that is complemented by the garlic and lemon, making this AIP-compliant side a must for your next big dinner!

Healing Autoimmune

AIP Chicken Lettuce Wraps

Ingredients: avocado oil, mushrooms, garlic, ginger, ground chicken, lemon juice, coconut aminos, iceberg lettuce leaves, spring onion, cilantro.

Lettuce wraps may be a new thing to you or you might be used to them by now, but whatever way they make a lovely quick and easy lunchtime dish. This recipe has a lot of Asian flavor because of the garlic, ginger and coconut aminos.

AIP Waldorf Salad

– Healing Autoimmune

AIP Waldorf Salad

Ingredients: coconut cream, lemon juice, salt, Granny Smith or another green apple, celery, grapes, romaine lettuce.

Waldorf salad is traditionally made with a creamy dressing and in this recipe this comes from the coconut cream and lemon juice which keep the dressing dairy free. Aside from the lettuce, this also has the fresh flavors of apple and celery, making this a lovely light and delicious salad to enjoy for lunch on a summer day, or as an appetizer for a dinner party. This is a simple recipe but it gives you a wonderfully tasty dish.

AIP Italian Burgers

– Healing Autoimmune

AIP Italian Burgers

Ingredients: ground beef, Italian seasoning, garlic powder, onion powder.

This is one of the simplest burger recipes out there and it is totally adaptable to any kind of eating plan. Sometimes simple is best – mix the meat and seasoning, form the patties and cook! A tasty meal ready in minutes! If the weather is not grilling-friendly, you can shallow fry these burgers indoors, but they make a lovely dish for a family barbecue!

AIP Chicken Salad Recipe With Grapes, Apple, and Celery

– Healing Autoimmune

AIP Chicken Salad Recipe With Grapes, Apple, and Celery

Ingredients: chicken breast, coconut oil, grapes, gala apple, celery, coconut milk, salt.

AIP chicken salads can be so much better when you add fruit! The grapes give the whole dish a juicy texture and there is a great crunch from the celery too. Adding the lemon juice also stops the apple from going brown, leaving your salad looking fresh and delicious. If you are not into celery you can always add shredded carrot instead.

Creamy AIP Mango Chicken Salad Recipe with Coconut Caesar Dressing

– Healing Autoimmune

Creamy AIP Mango Chicken Salad Recipe with Coconut Caesar Dressing

Ingredients: romaine lettuce, chicken breasts, coconut oil, mango, coconut cream, coconut oil, garlic or garlic powder, salt.

What a wonderful fusion of flavor and texture! You have meaty chicken, soft and sweet mango and a crunch from the celery, all tied together with a creamy dressing, which is reminiscent of traditional Caesar dressing. If you don't have fresh garlic you can just use garlic powder, and if you don't have mango you can use other fruits like peach or pineapple.

Smoked Salmon and Cucumber Ham Wraps

– Paleo Flourish

Smoked Salmon and Cucumber Ham Wraps

Ingredients: ham, cucumber, smoked salmon, coconut cream, green salad.

These tasty wraps are ideal for a lunchtime snack or even for a healthy breakfast. They have a lovely texture since all the layers are sandwiched together with the smooth coconut cream. These are easy to eat, so they would be perfect if you are feeding kids. Or why not try turning them inside out – make cucumber cups, chop the meat and stir in the cream and fill the cups with the mix to make dainty Paleo finger food!

Avocado Peach Prosciutto Salad

– Paleo Flourish

Paleo Avocado Peach Prosciutto Salad

Ingredients: peach, avocado, prosciutto, salad greens, lemon juice, extra virgin olive oil, sea salt.

This lovely paleo salad recipe is a great example of keeping things simple to bring out the flavor of the ingredients. You are only using oil and lemon to make the dressing and this will not detract from the flavors of the ham and fruit. As avocado and peach are both quite soft, it is a good idea to serve this with the prosciutto as a salty contrast in texture and flavor.

5 Ingredient Salmon Patties

– The Curious Coconut

5 Ingredient Salmon Patties

Ingredients: wild Alaskan pink salmon, canned pumpkin, coconut flour, tapioca starch, AIP-compliant pesto of choice, fat of choice.

Traditional fish cake recipes always seem to use egg to bind the mixture together, which can be a problem if you can't eat eggs. However this recipe uses pumpkin puree instead, which helps to hold the shape of the patties. They will still be easily broken, so try not to flip them any more than you have to. Note that pesto often contains pine nuts, which are not appropriate for strict AIP. Instead you can garnish with lemon wedges.

AIP Avocado Salad Recipe

– Healing Autoimmune

AIP Avocado Salad Recipe

Ingredients: red onion, red wine vinegar, avocado, salt, pickled beetroot, carrot, olive oil, chives.

This simple salad of creamy avocado, earthy beets, and pickled red onions is the perfect lunch fix. Make sure to pick a nice ripe avocado for this recipe and squeeze some lemon juice over it to stop it from browning. Beets are great for adding a bit of color to this salad, as well as a whole lot of important nutrients.

Easy AIP Recipes – Dinners

AIP Broccoli Soup

– Healing Autoimmune

AIP Broccoli Soup

Ingredients: broccoli, chicken broth/vegetable broth, coconut cream, salt, parsley.

Traditional broccoli soup can be thickened with flour, but this simple recipe uses coconut cream and that works just as well but keeps the dish AIP-friendly. This is a filling and nutritious soup that you can enjoy any time, but a warming plateful would make a lovely dinner on a chilly day.

AIP Bacon-Wrapped Salmon

– Healing Autoimmune

AIP Bacon-Wrapped Salmon

Ingredients: salmon, bacon, olive oil, tarragon, lemon wedges.

This recipe shows an amazing way to cook salmon by wrapping it in bacon, and this can look good, taste great and help stop the fish from drying out as there is a bit of fat from the bacon. This lovely AIP protein-packed dish would even make a good alternative to serve at Christmas or for a fancy dinner party.

AIP Baked Lemon Salmon

Ingredients: lemons, salmon filets, olive oil, salt, black pepper (omit), thyme sprigs, beetroot salad.

Those people who follow an autoimmune diet are usually doing it for health reasons, but they certainly don't have to rely on bland and boring food! This lemon salmon dish is so tasty and the citrus helps to cut through the fattiness of the fish really well. One tip – any leftovers make a great salad for tomorrow's lunch!

Many people believe that by changing their diet, they can affect their rheumatoid arthritis and better manage the disease. There are a lot of diets available, some more trendy than others. Should you be following the autoimmune protocol diet?

How to Control RA and Take Your Life Back

Does the Autoimmune Protocol Diet Help Rheumatoid Arthritis?

Many people believe that by changing their diet, they can affect their rheumatoid arthritis and better manage the disease. There are a lot of diets available, some more trendy than others. Should you be following the autoimmune protocol diet?

By Carol Eustice

Medically Reviewed by Alexa Meara, MD

Save

Sweet potatoes, chicken, and some vegetables can be part of an AIP diet.

Sweet potatoes, chicken, and some vegetables can be part of an AIP diet. Shutterstock

There's the gluten-free diet, ketogenic diet, vegan diet, Zone diet, South Beach diet, and more. If you listen to the news or are active on social media, you likely have heard of these diets and know people who tried them.

Among people with rheumatoid arthritis (RA), there is a popular notion that RA can be managed with diet, thereby skipping the undesirable side effects associated with certain medication. There is even an autoimmune protocol (AIP) diet, which by its name alone makes you think you should be on board.

In autoimmune diseases, the body mistakenly attacks its own tissues, causing damage. The autoimmune protocol diet works on inflammation in the gut, which is thought to be associated with autoimmune disease. Specifically, the AIP diet is thought to heal the immune system and the gut mucosa (lining), impacting inflammatory diseases, such as rheumatoid arthritis.

Is the AIP Diet the Same As the Paleo Diet?

The autoimmune protocol diet is considered the same as the Paleo diet by some. You will also see AIP called a "version" of the Paleo diet. Some say it is a stricter version of the Paleo diet. The principle behind the AIP diet is that autoimmune conditions are caused by "leaky gut" or altered intestinal permeability. In leaky gut, food leaks through tiny holes in the gut, provoking a response — actually an overreaction — by the immune system.

With the AIP diet, you eat foods that are rich in nutrients and steer clear of foods that are considered pro-inflammatory. Through diet, the goal is to not provoke an autoimmune response by the immune system. Summary of goals: Avoid irritating the gut with foods, heal holes in the gut, and reduce inflammation and other symptoms of autoimmune disease.

How the Autoimmune Protocol Diet Was Developed

The autoimmune protocol diet has been attributed to Loren Cordain, PhD, a scientist who discovered that certain foods can sometimes trigger inflammation in people with autoimmune disease. Author Robb Wolf outlined the autoimmune protocol in his book, The Paleo Solution, introducing it as an elimination diet. Sarah Ballantyne, PhD, (also known as The Paleo Mom) became interested in the autoimmune protocol, researched the science behind it, and wrote about it in her book, The Paleo Approach. Dr. Ballantyne is considered a leading expert on the autoimmune protocol.

Foods That Are Allowed and Disallowed on the Autoimmune Protocol Diet

The AIP diet allows you to eat:

Meat (preferably grass-fed) and fish

Vegetables, excluding nightshade vegetables

Sweet potatoes

Fruit in small quantities

Coconut milk

Avocado, olive, and coconut oil

Dairy-free fermented foods (examples: kombucha, sauerkraut, kefir made with coconut milk, kimchi)

Honey or maple syrup in small quantities

Fresh nonseed herbs (examples: basil, mint, oregano)

Green tea, and nonseed herbal teas

Bone broth

Vinegars

Grass-fed gelatin and arrowroot starch

The AIP diet does not allow you to eat:

All grains (including oats, wheat, and rice)

All dairy

Eggs

Nuts and seeds

Legumes and beans

Nightshade vegetables (tomatoes, potatoes, eggplant, peppers)

All sugars, including alternative sugars, such as stevia and xylitol

Butter and ghee (clarified butter)

Oils (other than coconut oil, olive oil, and avocado oil, which are allowed)

Herbs derived from seeds

Food additives or processed foods

Chocolate

Alcohol

Does the Autoimmune Protocol Diet Work for People With RA?

Researchers have been looking into the role of diet in leaky gut and autoimmune disease since at least 2012, and more current research suggests that, in some people, leaky gut may be linked to the development of autoimmune disease. But there are still no conclusive clinical studies with regard to the role of diet in leaky gut and autoimmune disease.

According to an article published in May 2014 in the journal FEBS Letters, "Rheumatoid arthritis is a multifactorial disease that involves both genetic and environmental factors. Among genetic factors, human leukocyte antigen (HLA) alleles provide the strongest risk, while among environmental factors, smoking and infections are involved. A role of hormones and changes in immune system during aging are also associated with pathogenesis of rheumatoid arthritis. All the factors that influence RA also impact the gut microbial composition. Gut microbiome provides a link between all the factors that influence RA. An individual may harbor a core gut microbiome and certain species may contract or expand depending on the exposure to various environmental factors, thus influencing the immune system locally in the gut as well as adaptive immune system."

There Appears to Be Gut Involvement in Rheumatoid Arthritis

But still, there is no specific diet that has been proven to help RA. The impact of diet on RA remains theoretical. It's trial-and-error at best. Essentially it's an elimination diet whereby you eliminate foods regarded as inflammatory and reintroduce them into your diet over time to see their effect on you individually. That's the best we have at this stage because nothing about diet has been proven to help RA patients collectively.

A small study published in November 2017 in the journal Inflammatory Bowel Diseases concluded that the autoimmune protocol can have an effect on inflammatory bowel disease (IBD). There were 15 patients with either Crohn's disease or ulcerative colitis enrolled in the study. They took six weeks to phase out the disallowed foods in the autoimmune protocol, followed by five weeks maintaining the protocol. Eleven of the 15 study participants had a complete remission. Great news for sure. But 15 is a very small study group — and there was no control group, and the study was not randomized. That said, to date this is the best clinical study we have for the autoimmune protocol diet. There is no such published study for RA. It's lacking and it's needed.

Autoimmune disease is an epidemic in our society, affecting an estimated 50 million Americans. But it doesn't have to be. Although genetic predisposition accounts for approximately one-third of your risk of developing an autoimmune disease, the other two-thirds comes from your environment, your diet, and your lifestyle. In fact, experts are increasingly recognizing that certain dietary factors are key contributors to autoimmune disease, placing these autoimmune conditions in the same class of diet- and lifestyle-related diseases as type 2 diabetes, cardiovascular disease, and obesity. This means that autoimmune disease is directly linked to our food choices and how we decide to live your life. It also means that we can manage and reverse autoimmune disease simply by changing how you eat and making more informed choices about sleep, activity, and stress... and that's some pretty darned good news!

There are more than one hundred confirmed autoimmune diseases and many more diseases that are suspected of having autoimmune origins (download a complete list here). The root cause of all autoimmune diseases is the same: our immune system, which is supposed to protect us from invading microorganisms, turns against us and attacks our proteins, cells, and tissues instead. Which proteins, cells, and tissues are attacked determines the autoimmune disease and its symptoms. In Hashimoto's thyroiditis, the thyroid gland is attacked. In rheumatoid arthritis, the tissues of your joints are attacked. In psoriasis, proteins within the layers of cells that make up your skin are attacked.

How does the immune system get so confused that it starts to attack our own bodies? It turns out that autoimmunity, the ability for the immune system to attack native tissues, is a relatively common accident. In fact, about 30% of people will have measurable levels of autoantibodies (antibodies that bind to some protein in our bodies instead of, or in addition to, a foreign protein, called an antigen) in their blood at any given time. In fact, this accident is so common, that our immune system has several failsafes for identifying autoimmunity and suppressing it. What occurs in autoimmune disease isn't just the accident of autoimmunity, but also failure of the immune system failsafes, stimulation of the immune system to attack, and the build up of enough damage in cells or tissues within the body to manifest as symptoms of a disease.

This confluence of events that culminates in autoimmune disease is a result of the interactions between your genes and your environment—a perfect storm of factors that cause the immune system to be unable to distinguish self (you) from invader (not you).

The Paleo Autoimmune Protocol, typically abbreviated AIP, is a powerful strategy that uses diet and lifestyle to regulate the immune system, putting an end to these attacks and giving the body the opportunity to heal.

The Autoimmune Protocol, abbreviated AIP, is a complementary approach to chronic disease management focused on providing the body with the nutritional resources required for immune regulation, gut health, hormone regulation and tissue healing while removing inflammatory stimuli from both diet and lifestyle. The AIP diet provides balanced and complete nutrition while avoiding processed and refined foods and empty calories. The AIP lifestyle encourages sufficient sleep, stress management and activity as these are important immune modulators.

Foods can be viewed as having two kinds of constituents within them: those that promote health (like nutrients!) and those that undermine health (like inflammatory compounds). (While there are constituents that neither promote nor undermine health, they are not used to evaluate the merit of an individual food.) Some foods are obvious wins for a health-promoting diet because they have tons of beneficial constituents and very few or no constituents that undermine health—good examples of these superfoods are organ meats, seafood, and most vegetables. Other foods are obvious fails because they have a relative lack of health-promoting constituents and are rife with problematic compounds—good examples are gluten-containing grains, peanuts, and most soy products. But many foods fall into the amorphous world of gray in between these two extremes. Tomatoes, for example, have some exciting nutrients, but they also contain several compounds that are so effective at stimulating the immune system that they have been investigated for use in vaccines as adjuvants (the chemicals in vaccines that enhance your immune response to whatever you're getting immunized against). The biggest difference between the Autoimmune Protocol and other dietary templates that take a nutrients-first approach while considering inflammation triggers is where we draw the line between "yes" foods and "no" foods in order to get more health-promoting compounds and fewer detrimental compounds in our diet. Those who are typically quite healthy can tolerate less-optimal foods than those who aren't. You can think of the Autoimmune Protocol as a pickier version of other evidence-based dietary templates; it accepts only those foods that are clear winners.

As such, the Autoimmune Protocol places greater emphasis on the most nutrient-dense foods in our food supply, including organ meat, seafood, and vegetables. And the Autoimmune Protocol eliminates foods endorsed by other healthy diets that have compounds that may stimulate the immune system or harm the gut environment, including nightshades (like tomatoes and peppers), eggs, nuts, seeds, and alcohol. The goal of the Autoimmune Protocol is to flood the body with nutrients while simultaneously avoiding any food that might be contributing to disease (or at the very least interfering with our efforts to heal).

The AIP is an elimination diet strategy, cutting out the foods that are most likely to be holding back our health. After a period of time, many of the excluded foods, especially those that have nutritional merit despite also containing some (but not too much) potentially detrimental compounds, can be reintroduced. The AIP is not a life sentence, but rather a toolbox full of strategies for understanding how your body reacts to foods, lifestyle and your environment and methodologies for healing given your individual health challenges.

The AIP is also a holistic approach to health, including not only a dietary framework but also a focus on lifestyle factors known to be important modulators of immune function, gut health, and hormone health. This includes a strong focus on getting adequate sleep, managing stress, and living an active lifestyle while avoiding overtraining. These three lifestyle factors are each essential for gut health because they directly influence the gut microbiome (getting enough sleep, keeping stress levels in check, and being active are all essential for a healthy and diverse gut microbial community in addition to supporting the growth of key probiotic strains). Chronic stress and overtraining also increase intestinal permeability. Sleep, stress and activity are all essential hormone modulators; for example, insulin sensitivity is more strongly influenced by these lifestyle factors than it is by diet. And, most importantly, immune function is directly tied to lifestyle. Inflammation is triggered by getting inadequate less, feeling stressed, being sedentary, and overtraining. Furthermore, the regulatory aspects of the immune system are most active while we're sleeping, and sleep quality is linked to stress. Additionally, there's emerging evidence that a strong sense of connection and community as well as spending time in natural environments also contribute to a healthier immune system.

Drawing on insights gleaned from more than 1,200 scientific studies, the AIP is now supported by clinical trial evidence.

In a 2017 study, fifteen patients with active inflammatory bowel disease were placed on the Autoimmune Protocol by transitioning gradually over 6 weeks, followed by a 5-week maintenance phase. Patients were closely monitored and given access to health coaching. They were also given two books The Paleo Approach by Dr. Sarah Ballantyne, PhD (which remains the definitive AIP guidebook) and The Autoimmune Wellness Handbook by Mickey Trescott, NTP and Angie Alt, NTC, CHC, as resources for following the protocol. Clinical remission was achieved by week 6 (yes, just by completing the transition to the AIP) in eleven of the fifteen participants (73%!!), and they stayed in remission throughout the 5-week maintenance phase of the study. All patients, including those that didn't achieve clinical remission, experienced quantifiable improvement in disease activity over the entire course of the study. In a similarly-designed 2019 study, seventeen women with Hashimoto's thyroiditis were placed on the Autoimmune Protocol by transitioning gradually over 6 weeks, followed by a 4-week maintenance phase. Patients experienced a statistically significant improvement in health-related quality of life scores as measured by the 36-Item Short Form Health Survey and Cleveland Clinic Center for Functional Medicine's Medical Symptoms Questionnaire (MSQ). In fact, the clinical symptom burden, as measured by the MSQ, decreased from an average of 92 at the beginning of the study to 29 after the 10 weeks. This was accompanied by statistially significant reductions in C-reactive protein (a measurement of systemic inflammation) and white blood cell counts

Following the AIP diet involves increasing your intake of nutrient-dense, health-promoting foods while avoiding foods that may be triggers for your disease.

In summary, the rules of what to eat are:

organ meat and offal (aim for 5 times per week, the more the better)–read more here.

fish and shellfish (wild is best, but farmed is fine) (aim for at least 3 times per week, the more the better)–read more here and here.

vegetables of all kinds, as much variety as possible and the whole rainbow, aim for 8+ servings daily

Leafy green vegetables (lettuce, spinach, kale, collards, celery leaves, etc.)

Colorful vegetables and fruit (red, purple, blue, yellow, orange, white)

Cruciferous vegetables (broccoli, cabbage, kale, turnips, arugula, cauliflower, Brussels sprouts, watercress, mustard greens, etc.)

Roots, tubers and winter quash (cassava, sweet potato, parsnip, beets, fennel, carrots, rutabaga, turnip, acorn squash, spaghetti squash, etc.)

Onion family (aka alliums, onions, leek, garlic, ramps, etc.)

Sea vegetables (excluding algae like chlorella and spirulina which are immune stimulators)

Mushrooms (and other edible fungi)

herbs and spices

quality meats (grass-fed, pasture-raised, wild as much as possible) (poultry in moderation due to high omega-6 content unless you are eating a ton of fish)

healthy fats (pasture-raised/grass-fed animal fats [rendered or as part of your meat], fatty fish, olive oil, avocado oil, coconut oil, palm oil[not palm kernel])

fruit (keeping fructose intake between 10g and 40g daily-note that 20g is probably optimal)

probiotic/fermented foods (fermented vegetables or fruit, kombucha, water kefir, coconut milk kefir, coconut milk yogurt, supplements)–read about them here and here.

glycine-rich foods (anything with connective tissue, joints or skin, organ meat, and bone broth)

gut microbiome superfoods (high-fiber and phytonutrient fruits and vegetables, cruciferous vegetables, mushrooms, roots, tubers, alliums, leafy greens, berries, apple family, citrus, extra virgin olive oil, fish, shellfish, honey and bee products, fermented foods, edible insects, tea, and bone broth)

Source the best-quality ingredients you can.

Eat as much variety as possible

In addition, remove the following from your diet:

Grains

Legumes

Dairy

Refined and processed sugars and oils

Eggs (especially the whites)

Nuts (including nut butters, flours and oils)

Seeds (including seed oil, cocoa, coffee and seed-based spices)

Nightshades (potatoes [sweet potatoes are fine], tomatoes, eggplants, sweet and hot peppers, cayenne, red pepper, tomatillos, goji berries etc. and spices derived from peppers, including paprika)

Potential Gluten Cross-Reactive Foods

Alcohol

NSAIDS (like aspirin or ibuprofen)

Non-nutritive sweeteners (yes, all of them, even stevia and monk fruit)

Emulsifiers, thickeners, and other food additives

Moderate your intake of the following:

Fructose (from fruits and starchy vegetables, aiming for between 10g and 40g daily-note that 20g is probably optimal)

Salt (using only unrefined salt such as Himalayan pink salt or Celtic gray salt)

High-glycemic-load fruits and vegetables (such as dried fruit, plantain, and taro root) – note, the AIP is not low-carb (see The Case for More Carbs: Insulin's Non-Metabolic Roles in the Human Body)

Omega-6 polyunsaturated fatty acid–rich foods (such as poultry and fatty cuts of industrially produced meat)

Black and green tea (up to 3-4 cups per day is okay for most people)

Coconut

Natural sugars (honey and blackstrap molasses are the best choice)

Saturated fat (aiming for 10-15% of total calories)

This diet is appropriate for everyone with diagnosed autoimmune disorders or with suspected autoimmune diseases. It is very simply an extremely nutrient-dense diet that is devoid of foods that irritate the gut, cause gut dysbiosis and activate the immune system. You will not be missing out on any nutrients and this diet is absolutely appropriate to follow for the rest of your life. If you have a specific autoimmune disease that causes extra food sensitivities, those should be taken into account with your food choices.

Lifestyle Factors

Don't forget the crucial importance of: getting enough sleep (at least 8-10 hours every night), managing stress (mindful meditation is very well studied in the scientific literature and universally shown to be beneficial), protecting circadian rhythms (being outside during the day, being in the dark at night and avoiding bright lights in the evening), enjoying nature, nurturing social connection, having fun, making time for hobbies, relaxing, and getting lots of mild to moderately intense activity (while avoiding intense/strenuous activity). Read more about the Paleo lifestyle here.

Take a few hours on the weekend to prep meals

I love to take a few hours on Sunday, and maybe 1-2 hours during the middle of the week to batch cook. Not only do I go into the week feeling prepared, but I save hours in the kitchen throughout the week by doing it all at once!

This takes time to get used to, but I promise, it's a huge time saver!

The freezer is your friend!

Don't want to eat the same meals throughout the week? Throw some of your meal prep into the freezer so you can easily rotate different foods in and out of your diet.

Unbound Wellness

BREAKFAST SAUSAGE CHICKEN POPPERS (PALEO, WHOLE 30, AIP)

These breakfast sausage chicken poppers are the perfect breakfast option with veggies, protein, and flavor in one bite! They're paleo, whole30, and AIP.

chicken sausage poppers on a plate

BREAKFAST SAUSAGE CHICKEN POPPERS

Who doesn't love breakfast sausage? Most conventional sausages are made with nightshade spices (which I don't tolerate), unwanted fillers, or just aren't the best quality. That's why I created these Breakfast Sausage Sweet Potato Chicken Poppers have all of the flavor and none of the unwanted junk!

These sausage patties aren't your average breakfast. In just one little popper, you get a sweet potato, spinach, apple, bacon, and flavorful herbs! So good and full of flavor, you don't even need a maple syrupy sauce.

THE INGREDIENTS FOR THE BREAKFAST SAUSAGE CHICKEN POPPERS

Sweet potato. I use a large grater to grate the sweet potato, but you can also use a food processor.

Ground chicken. You can also use ground turkey, or simply use the food processor to grind chicken breast or thighs!

Spinach.

Apple. I use gala or a honey crisp, or granny smith apple, but you can get away with using what you have on hand!

Bacon. I like the applegate brand.

Coconut flour. This is used a binder. You can also use other flours like almond or cassava flour.

Coconut oil. Or you can use olive or avocado oil!

These breakfast sausage chicken poppers are the perfect breakfast option with veggies, protein, and flavor in one bite! They're paleo, whole30, and AIP.

chicken sausage poppers on a plate

BREAKFAST SAUSAGE CHICKEN POPPERS

Who doesn't love breakfast sausage? Most conventional sausages are made with nightshade spices (which I don't tolerate), unwanted fillers, or just aren't the best quality. That's why I created these Breakfast Sausage Sweet Potato Chicken Poppers have all of the flavor and none of the unwanted junk!

These sausage patties aren't your average breakfast. In just one little popper, you get a sweet potato, spinach, apple, bacon, and flavorful herbs! So good and full of flavor, you don't even need a maple syrupy sauce.

THE INGREDIENTS FOR THE BREAKFAST SAUSAGE CHICKEN POPPERS

Sweet potato. I use a large grater to grate the sweet potato, but you can also use a food processor.

Ground chicken. You can also use ground turkey, or simply use the food processor to grind chicken breast or thighs!

Spinach.

Apple. I use gala or a honey crisp, or granny smith apple, but you can get away with using what you have on hand!

Bacon. I like the applegate brand.

Coconut flour. This is used a binder. You can also use other flours like almond or cassava flour.

Coconut oil. Or you can use olive or avocado oil!

Chicken breast sausage ingredients in a bowl

HOW TO MAKE BREAKFAST SAUSAGE CHICKEN POPPERS

Take the raw sweet potato and squeeze it with a paper towel or cheesecloth to remove any excess liquid.

Using a large mixing bowl, combine all of the ingredients and mix well.

Roll the poppers. Begin rolling the mixture into small poppers about one inch in diameter (you'll have about 20-25 poppers) and slightly flatten each of them with the palm of your hand. Place them on the baking sheet

Bake in the oven for 25-28 minutes, flipping halfway through. If desired, crisp further in a pan or place under the broiler if desired for 1-2 minutes.

Remove from the oven when thoroughly cooked through and the internal temperature reads 165 F.

Allow to cool and serve immediately, or store in the fridge or freezer as a make-ahead breakfast!

CAN YOU MAKE THESE AHEAD OF TIME?

Yes! These are so perfect for meal prep! I make them ahead of time and store them in the fridge for up to 3-4 days.

CAN YOU FREEZE THESE?

Yes! They freeze great! I would recommend cooking them first and them freezing them afterwards.

CAN YOU FRY THEM IN A PAN INSTEAD OF BAKE THEM?

I haven't tried that, but it should work!

WHAT CAN YOU SERVE WITH THEM?

I think they're a great meal on their own, but you can also have a side

INGREDIENTS

1 lb ground chicken (or turkey)

1 cup shredded sweet potato

1/2 cup spinach, finely chopped

1/2 cup apple, finely diced

2-3 slices of bacon, finely diced

2 tbsp coconut oil

2 tbsp coconut flour

1 tsp ground sage

1/2 tsp sea salt

1 tsp rosemary

INSTRUCTIONS

Preheat the oven to 400 F and line a baking sheet with parchment paper

Take the raw sweet potato and squeeze it with a paper towel or cheesecloth to remove any excess liquid.

Using a large mixing bowl, combine all of the ingredients and mix well.

Begin rolling the mixture into small poppers about one inch in diameter (you'll have about 20-25 poppers) and slightly flatten each of them with the palm of your hand. Place them on the baking sheet

Bake in the oven for 25-28 minutes, flipping halfway through. If desired, crisp further in a pan or place under the broiler if desired for 1-2 minutes.

Remove from the oven when thoroughly cooked through and the internal temperature reads 165 F.

Allow to cool and serve immediately, or store in the fridge or freezer as a make-ahead breakfast!

MEXICAN BREAKFAST SKILLET

Unbound Wellness

Eggs are such a staple for breakfasts, and were probably one of the only real foods that I ate as a kid. Who doesn't love scrambled eggs for breakfast or a hard boiled egg for a quick snack? They're easy, convenient, and nutrient dense… but so many people (myself included) have egg sensitivities and allergies! The question arises "what are you supposed to eat for breakfast if you're egg free?!". Breakfast is one of the hardest meals if you're egg free, on the autoimmune protocol or just egg free on a paleo or Whole30 type diet. So I'm adding to my egg free breakfast recipes with this Mexican Breakfast Skillet! It's Paleo, AIP, Whole30, and the perfect egg free breakfast.

When I announced that I was doing a Whole30 (I'm on day 6 right now!!) during February/March, I was asked "why the heck do you need a Whole30 if you're already Paleo and mostly AIP?". Main answer... treats! There are tons of recipes for AIP treats (I have plenty of my own!) and I was really feeling like I needed a break. My second reason was to show you guys how you can do Whole30 mostly AIP! No eggs, no nuts, no nightshades, and no premade bars. So an egg free breakfast dish was one of my top priorities to share with you!

This Mexican Breakfast Skillet is such an amazing and balanced breakfast. It feature green veggies, a starchy veggie, healthy protein, and healthy fat, to keep you satiated throughout the day, and much less likely to experience blood sugar spikes and dips.

WHAT YOU NEED FOR THIS MEXICAN BREAKFAST SKILLET

Ground beef

Grass-fed ground beef was my protein of choice for this skillet, but you can also use something like turkey, chicken or even compliant chorizo... I just think beef provides the best flavor here!

Sweet potato

The starchy veggie of choice in this skillet.

Kale, red onion, radish, and cilantro

These veggies add nutrient density, and tons of flavor to the dish.

Avocado

What would a taco skillet be without avocado??

Optional : Salsa, or fried eggs

As this dish is AIP, it's nightshade free and egg free. However, if you can tolerate salsa and eggs, go for it!

Mexican Breakfast Skillet (Paleo, Whole30, AIP, Egg Free)

INGREDIENTS

1 lb ground beef

2 medium sweet potatoes, diced

1 medium red onion, finely diced

2 stalks kale, destemmed and chopped

2 tsp cumin (omit for AIP)

2 tsp dried oregano

2 tsp garlic powder

2 tsp onion powder

1 tsp sea salt

1/2 tsp black pepper (omit for AIP)

Juice of one lime

For garnish

2 tbsp cilantro, chopped

1-2 radishes, sliced

1 medium avocado

Optional

Fresh salsa

INSTRUCTIONS

Set the stove top to medium heat and prepare a large skillet

Add the ground beef to the pan and lightly salt. Cook on medium heat until browned, and set aside, reserving most of the fat in the pan to cook the vegetables.

Add the sweet potatoes and cook until softened and crisped (but not burnt), stirring frequently

Next add in the red onion and cook until the onions are translucent

Finally, add the kale and cook for 2-3 minutes or until wilted

Add back in the beef, as well as the salt, pepper, cumin, oregano, onion powder, garlic, lime juice and stir for until well combined

To serve, top with avocado, cilantro, and radish

Eat as a breakfast skillet, or lunch leftovers!